Also by Dr. Stenbeck

Available from the usual on-line source

Books
Healing Yourself -- The Holistic Approach
   [An introduction to Holistic Self-healing.]

Heal Yourself Right Now!
   [The Seven Priority Organ Levels for
      effective Nutritional/Holistic Treatment of
      all organs.]

The 22 Unique Body Types
   (for Health and Weight Loss)

Q & A to Identify Your Body Type (Booklet)
   [Individual Type booklets are also available

Booklets
(Step-by-step instructions on healing yourself)

   #1 Start Healing with Positive Thinking
   #2 Mastering Positive Feelings for Health!
   #3 Spiritual Balance and Your Healing

The Calciferic Body Type

Representing one of the 22 Body Types first described by Victor Rocine around 1900

The Abraham Lincoln, Robin Wright Celebrity Body Type

For Kaye,
there at the beginning with Doc Severn,
and for Liberty,
continuing the holistic healing journey…

Disclaimer

The information in this book is for educational purposes only and is not a substitute for medication, diets, or other medical care. The diets do not treat diseases or medical conditions, and are an adjunct to your orthodox health care.

The author and publisher accept no responsibility for any misuse of the information within. If you have any physical problem, food allergy, emotional disorder, or disease, common sense dictates that you consult with a physician before changing your diet, taking nutritional supplements, or following the advice given here.

———

About the Author

Educated in New Zealand and in the U.S.A., Dr. Stenbeck attained B.Sc. (NZ), M.S., and D.C. degrees. His holistic healing methods have been profiled in magazines (Esquire, McLean's, Playgirl, the Atlanta Constitution), and on TV in the USA and in Canada. He was the main contributor to the Warner Book, _The Eye/Body Connection_ by Jessica Maxwell that focused on the holistic healing relationships between the iris structure and organ genetics.

In the 1970-80's he was elected Fellow, Royal Society of Health, London; Fellow, American Association of Chemists; Member, American Association of Clinical Chemists; and Affiliate, Royal Society of Medicine, London. He studied naturopathy and Body Types with Dr. Bernard Jensen and Dr. Clifford Severn, and has practiced in medical partnerships where patients received the joint benefits of medical and holistic healing.

He is a member of Self-Realization Fellowship. To receive advice on any health issue from a holistic viewpoint, or to receive help with your body type, see his web site: *DrStenbeck.net*

———

Contents

* * *

The Calciferic Body Type and Food Guide

Appendix

The 22 Body Types:
Celebrity Examples

---

*This Booklet contains the **Calciferic** type. See The 22 Unique Body Types for all type descriptions.]*

———

Thin Types

Atrophic	*Woody Allen / Audrey Hepburn*
	Stan Laurel / Calista Flockheart
Exesthesic	*Cher / Sarah Jessica Parker*
	(Female type only)
Marasmic	*President Obama / Princess Diana*
	James Stewart / Kate Blanchard
Neurogenic	*J.K. Simmons / Joan Rivers*
	Jon Cryer / Marin Hinle
Pathoferic	*(No celebrity males)*
	Blythe Danner / Gwyneth Paltrow
Sillevitic	*David Bowie / Shirley MacLaine*
	Rod Stewart / Carol Channing

Muscle Types

Calciferic	*Michael Jordan / Angelica Huston* *Abraham Lincoln / Robin Wright*
Carbogenic	*George Clooney / Lady Gaga* *Pres. G. Bush, Jr. / Meg Ryan*
Desmogenic	*Marlon Brando / Loni Anderson* *Daniel Craig / Tina Turner*
Eldic	*Ross Perot / Hillary Clinton* *Peter Falk / Sigourney Weaver*
Medeic	*Gary Oldman / Madonna* *John Hurt / Marlene Deitrich*
Myogenic	*Pres. Bill Clinton / Sharon Stone* *Pres. John Kennedy / Julia Roberts*
Nervimotive	*Frank Sinatra / Elizabeth Taylor* *Mark Wahlbberg / Natalie Wood*
Nitropheric	*Ben Affleck / Ava Gardner* *Kirk Douglas / Kate Winslet*
Pallinomic	*Pres. Donald Trump /* *Attorney General Janet Reno* *Bill O'Reilly (Fox) / Jane Russell*

Fat Types

Barotic   *Robin Williams / 'Mrs.Doubtfire'*
                 Elton John / William Conrad

Carboferic   *Bill Murray / Roseanne*
                 Billy Gardell / Melissa McCarthy

Hydripheric   *John Goodman / Shelly Winters*
                 Wayne Knight / Jennifer Holliday

Isogenic   *Einstein / Oprah Winfrey*
                 Phillip S .Hoffman / Queen Victoria

Lipopheric   *Rush Limbaugh / Rosie O'Donnell*
                 Chris Christie / Camryn Manheim

Oxypheric   *Winston Churchill / Orsen Welles*
                 Ella Fitzgerald / Gerry Spence

Pargenic   *Burt Reynolds / Katey Segal*
                 Ron Perlman / Kirstey Alley

Dr.Lloyd Stenbeck

Succinct Quote on Human Types

From Victor Rocine, who first described discrete body types around 1900.

"A type is an order of people that differentiates and distinguishes itself by a general and similar form, brain-formation, chemistry, structure, build, immunity, tendencies, predisposition, resemblance, skin-pigment, and type characteristics based on observation and analogy.

"Or, in other words, people of a given type are similar physically and like-minded as if they were brothers and sisters—that is what type means.

"Everything in nature is made according to plan. Man only discovers that plan and gives it a name. The zoologist has not made the animals—he has only described the plan adopted by the wonderful Creator, and named the classes, sub-classes, etc.

"How important type research will be to humanity, time alone will make known."

———

Prologue

The esteemed scientist J. J. Berzelius, discoverer of several chemical elements, inspired Victor Rocine to research body types and to investigate the correlation between types and their diseases. Around 1890-1910, Rocine privately published his original findings on the mineral basis of different body types, and this present book exists because of his brilliant insights.

For many years, I studied with Dr. Clifford Severn who had been a personal student of Victor Rocine on body types, naturopathy, herbology, iris analysis, diet, and nutritional healing methods. He had a successful career as a lecturer and healer, and was one of those rare athletes with complete muscle control over his body. I saw him under a spotlight at 85 years of age, contracting and rippling every individual muscle in his perfectly developed body. Field-Marshal Jan Smuts, the WWII South African Prime Minister, devoted a full chapter of his autobiography to how Severn's healing methods had saved his life. In the 1950's, *Life* magazine did a four-page spread on Severn and his family. Fame he had.

Another Rocine student I studied with, Dr. Bernard Jensen wrote of Rocine's body type research and nutritional methods in his privately published book <u>*The Chemistry of Man*</u>.

This book is deeply rooted in Rocine's original work, and with that of Herbert Shelton, M.D., Ph.D. (at Harvard University in the 1930's). I integrated their research with newer dietary and nervous system data along with celebrity examples of each type, hopefully, making this material easier to digest and more entertaining for the reader.

Gayelord Hauser, another Rocine student I knew, was a celebrated health book author. He wrote a popular book on Rocine's types in the 1940's, <u>*Types and Temperaments;*</u> reputedly, he also introduced yogurt to the western world.

This book exists because of Rocine's creative brilliance and original discoveries in natural healing.

▶ *Rocine: "The soul creates the body type."*

Rocine taught that the soul chooses a body type and brain to live in, thus presenting different experiences and life lessons to master. Why were *you* born the way you are?

That is something to think about, especially if it is true! What would your soul purpose be to live in a particular body type. I provide some thoughts on this issue in each type description and try to assess from my experience with your type the particular lessons of life presented therein.

Rocine was as brilliant in his way as an Abraham Lincoln, Michael Jordan, Michael Phelps, Tony Robbins, or a Daniel Day Lewis—all *calciferic* types—rare, leaders, innovative, brilliant, and highly intelligent in their different fields of endeavor.

Celebrity examples exist for most types, not a duplicate of you, but someone who has your essence in their body-mind individuality. Knowing your type allows you to become a better you!

The celebrity examples provide further help in identifying your body type.

▶ *Rocine's classic findings are the backbone of this book. Integrated with Sheldon's research and with other dietary and food issues including mental, emotional, and spiritual attributes,*

Many people take nutritional supplements and try different diets without a doctor's advice. If this is your choice, use common sense, listen to body responses, and discontinue any allergic reactions to foods or nutritional substances.

———

The Calciferic Body Type

* * *

"You may also have a physical or psychological feature not representative of your type such as height, weight, appearance, talent, weakness, strength, etc., due to biochemical errors, environmental influences, racial or cultural differences, and congenital or genetic issues. Nevertheless, the type identification of the average person is usually clear."

— *Victor Rocine*

Calciferic Type
Celebrity Examples

If you think this is your type, be sure to look at **on-line photographs** *of these examples. Look for general similarities to yourself. Note that sub-types cause the differences in appearance between members of the same type. This is a <u>very rare</u> type, as you will discern from the celebrities below. We know you as celebrities, but are highly unlikely to know you in everyday society.*

———

A spectacular list of famous and talented people!

GOVERNMENT

President Abraham Lincoln
President Andrew Jackson
President de Gaulle
Prime Minister Pierre Trudeau (Canada)
Prime Minister Margaret Thatcher (the
  "Iron lady" of Britain)

ACTORS

Daniel Day Lewis
James Coburn
Lee Marvin
John Huston

George MacReady (General in "Paths of
  Glory")
Sir Aubrey Smith (Black and white movies]

Robin Wright   Angelica Huston
Brigitte Nielsen   Grace Jones

In many of these actor's roles, their
forcefulness, command, authority, and grim
fortitude is evident.

SPORTS

Michael Phelps   Michael Jordan
Dwayne Johnson   Nick Kyrgios
Kobe Bryant

ARTS/OTHER

Andreas Seppi   Tony Robbins
Howard Stern
George Bernard Shaw

HISTORY

Charles Darwin (from Rocine)
Alexander the Great (from Rocine)
Sir Edmund Hillary (Mt. Everest conqueror
  from N.Z.)
Sir Keith Park (WWII Battle of Britain
  leader from N.Z.)

Lord Hugh Trenchard (WW1 General and "Father of the Royal Air Force")
AND...Victor Rocine himself

[Note: I knew two of the above celebrities, several brilliant scientists, which helped me identify their type and to know them very well.]

You already know something about this type from their public persona and appearance, whether from seeing them yourself or from the celebrity examples. You blend such insights with the type descriptions and the types of your family and friends, to discern their presence in your midst!

Read the types and if still confused you may like to use the personal request for type identification from my web site: *DrStenbeck.net*

———

Calciferic Type Questionnaire

These questions describe the generic type, and not specifically you! If any question ever applied to you, then choose the True answer!

For Question 1 only:

A = True	B = Maybe	C = Untrue
15 points	7 points	1 point

1. Physically identify with celebrity example ____

Then ...

A = True	B = Maybe	C = Untrue
5 points	3 points	1 point

---

2. Height is close to:
   Males: 6'2-7'0+   Females: 5'6-6'9+   ____
3. Usual weight is close to:
   Males: 185-280   Females 160-220   ____
4. Slender-medium-bony body, very tall,
   broad shoulders   ____
5. Compact, resilient strong muscles   ____
6. Weight controlled until middle-age   ____
7. Commanding presence, great poise,
   impressive posture   ____
8. Hair sparse, thin, balding with aging   ____
9. Face has prominent cheek-bones and
   sunken cheeks; the skin is tightly-lined   ____

10. Mentally original, creative, brilliant _____
11. Poised with good posture _____
12. Teeth large, strong, irregular shape with aging _____
13. Assertive, very aggressive, and combative (if provoked) _____
14. Calm and peaceful unless pushed too far, then they lay down the law _____
15. Appear grim, stern, threatening; are tame and docile unless provoked _____
16. If angered by someone, one day the score will be settled! _____
17. Strongly idealist, desire to help others to achieve their goals _____
18. Are orators, but dislike socializing with lesser minds _____
19. If in love, never stop pursuing until they win _____
20. Work and achieve goals through dedicated efforts _____
21. Have little time for the arts (or other right brain activities) _____
22. Have a giant left-brain for analyzing, assessing, rationalizing, thinking, and then taking dynamic action! _____
23. From under the eyes a facial line often reaches to the lower jaw _____
24. Have strong willpower; the mind is under control of powerful reason and will (more than other types) _____
25. Powerful intellect, debating power _____
26. Great tenacity and perseverance _____

27. Talented in science, mathematics, research, invention, speech, military, the objective world (and sports!) _____
28. Always prepared for future problems _____
29. Great objectivity: do not rely on faith, trust, beliefs or sentiments; are only interested in the facts _____
30. Slow to make friendships; friends must be intellectually worthy _____
31. History or tendency to arthritis, bone, or joint pain _____
32. Authoritative, strict with discipline _____
33. Highly moral and ethical _____
34. Face becomes deep red when upset _____
35. Genius-like _____
36. Serious and thoughtful _____
37. Respect rational intelligent people (have no time for others) _____
38. Males ruggedly handsome; females sternly attractive _____
39. Take command in emergencies; born warriors and leaders; the last to fall in battle _____
40. Learn from worldly experience rather than from books; if university trained, are innovative and brilliant _____
41. Lead by example and brilliance _____
42. Forehead large, prominent, square _____
43. Cynical, skeptical, and pessimistic; are never defeatist _____
44. Larger ears, set close to the head _____

45. Wide mouth; lips tend to be beup or down at one end, thin or thick, etc. _____
46. Large nostrils and bony nose _____
47. Voice strong, forceful, emphatic, arsh, commanding _____
48. Notably flat chest front to back; bust is small to moderate _____
49. Back bony, muscular _____
50. When healthy, flat abdomen, may distend with age; wide hip bones and a powerful pelvis _____
51. Long, bony, heavy, strong, muscular extremities; shoulders broad and bony, hands and feet large, bony; toes large _____
52. Premeditated severe, relentless justice; able to be vindictive _____
53. Strong sexual drive and performance _____

▶ *The type questionnaire pinpoints the major features of that type: if the celebrity examples are unhelpful, you may be an unusual variant (in which case ignore the celebrity issue and give yourself 7 points on Question 1).*

_____

Scoring

For question #1:

A response: give 15 points = _____

B response: give 7 points = _____

C response: give 1 points = _____

For questions #2—53:

A response: give 5 points = _____

B response: give 3 points = _____

C response: give 1 point = _____

Total of the above points = _____

Interpretation

138—255: PROBABLY Calciferic type

71—137: POSSIBLY Calciferic type

<71: NOT Calciferic type

The Calciferic Type

Rocine: "Calciferic means lime or calcium carrying." You utilize and hold more calcium in your tissues than any other type. You are the calcium type.

———

Y ou are a very rare person. Your type is always tall and muscular, well-built and strong. Some of you become heavy with age, but most stay medium-sized. You think slowly and ponderously, are deliberate, serious, thoughtful, honest, stern, sometimes dangerous looking, and tame and docile until aroused—then look out!

▶ *Rocine: "When angered you move swiftly to vengeance; when in love, there is no escape; in war, you show no mercy. You deliver cruel justice: premeditated, unforgiving, severe, relentless, and tenacious."*

You are born to be bold and heroic. Three famed New Zealanders are of your type: the conqueror of Everest, and two of the Royal Air Force leaders of WWII. You learn from worldly experience rather than from books, yet if university trained you are innovative and brilliant: a potential genius in war, science, government, invention, and philosophy. You are men and women of daring, action, and tenacity: Presidents Andrew Jackson, Abraham Lincoln, Charles De Gaulle, Charles Darwin, and Alexander the Great were your type. Note that British Royalty has knighted many of you for services to science, the arts, and the military.

▶ *Rocine: "Before believing anything you should see the objective truth with your giant left brain—you have little faith, trust, subjectivity, or metaphysical beliefs."*

You are like the ox: stubborn, slow, awkward, patient, and passive. In emergencies, you take command! If male, you shake your bald head, clench your bony fists, and take appropriate action. You are a born warrior, leader, and general: slow to take up arms and the last to fall.

You love work, endurance, effort, and more effort—you never give up! You are opposite to the *carboferic* who loves leisure, pleasure, and ease.

▶ *Rocine: "You are slow to anger but when up and going there is no stopping you. Ranting and raving, you give out a constant stream of orders, about which you are invariably right!"*

This is how Rocine describes himself:

"He is a man of strength, hardihood, endurance. He has an iron constitution, an iron will, iron mind. He is resolute, determined, grim, and sturdy. He has masculine attributes, iron nerves, hard bones, compact muscles, a strong fist, and a stiff spine. He is a man of accomplishments, daring, reason and insight…"

[And he goes on and on. Without a doubt, the rare calciferic type has a magnificent brain and ego.]

Physical Similarity to Other Types

The marasmic type (President H. W. Bush, Sr., Princess Diana) look somewhat similar, but is less grim and stern looking, more approachable, friendly (and psychologically the opposite).

The atrophic type (Tony Perkins) is leaner, non-aggressive, and more friendly.

———

Average Height and Weight

Males:	6'2-7'0+	185-280 pounds
Females:	5'6-6'9+	160-220 pounds

———

Calciferic Type Description

The calciferic type description represents how you appear in everyday society. You may have a sub-type that alters parts of this description.

Think of the celebrity examples as you read the descriptions. You are lean, bony, broad-shouldered, muscular, very strong, a flat body, and always tall. Your face and skin are tight, lined, and emaciated-looking with deep cheek indentations especially in males like Michael Jordan, James Coburn, and Howard Stern. You look older than you are. You have impressive poise and posture with somewhat awkward gestures. Although your stern face is not inviting, you are friendlier than appearances first suggest.

▶ *Rocine: "A great many calcium men are found among the Scotch and Swedes, and among Americans of the pioneer type."*
[Written around 1900]

Head — A large, prominent, square, and often retreating forehead is usually deeply furrowed in the males (who spend most of their time thinking and planning). The upper-central head is high and roof-shaped; your back-head is smaller.

Hair — Your hair is thin and falls easily, with most males showing balding by age 40-50 (unless you have a sub-type with prolific hair growth). The hair is coarse, black, or fair, with some early graying. The older males look ruggedly handsome (in their gray-white toupees).

Eyes — Typically, blue or gray eyes appear dull, threatening, and uninviting.

Ears — Larger and longer ears positioned close to the back head (unlike the male *eldic* type whose ears are large and sometimes floppy).

Nose — You have a large straight nose and nostrils.

Face — You commonly develop indented sunken cheeks, with a distinct line from under the eyes down to the lower jaw (as in Howard Stern and James Coburn). When upset your face takes on a deep red color.

Mouth and Lips —Your mouth is always wide, the lips rarely proportional or shapely, either being up or down at one end, or thin or thick. The upper lip is usually long, thin, and drawn; the lower lip is long, full, and often blood-filled. Your voice is strong, urging, forceful, deep, harsh, abrupt, and commanding. You demand attention!

Teeth — Usually large strong teeth, irregular, yellowing with age.

Skin — Your skin is variable in texture and color.

Neck —The neck is lean and long, strong and muscular.

Muscles — You are very strong and superb professional athletes (Michael Jordan), but unlike these athletes you rarely get excited about exercise systems; aerobics, light exercises, deep massage, horseback riding, and swimming benefit your health.

Chest — There is a notably flat chest from front to back (gorilla-like) in contrast to the *oxypheric and barotic* types (barrel-chested). The bust is small to moderate-sized (or larger if overweight).

Back and Shoulders — A long bony muscular back with broad-shoulders, and very visible shoulder blades.

Abdomen and Hips — Your abdomen is flat when health, but may distend with age, poor diet, and lack of exercise. The hips and pelvis are powerfully developed.

Arms and Legs — Long, bony, heavy, strong, lean, and muscular extremities; thick palms with large fingers, bony feet and toes are usual.

Joints — The bones and joints are strong, compact, and enduring.

Weight — You commonly gain up to 30 pounds with age and inactivity. Weight loss is easy with restricted calorie intake.

———

Calciferic Personality Traits

If you are this type many, but not all, of the following characteristics are present—you may have overcome or moderated the negatives, but recognize that you once had several of them.

You may have any of the following traits:

- Brilliant and unbeatable in intellectual debate
- Serious, solemn, deep thinking, self-actualizing
- High will power, controlling attitude, combative
- Patient, reliable, ethical, honest, and provocative
- Moral, honorable, ethical, passionate, and proud
- Great fighters: may be killed, but never conquered

▶ *Rocine: "You are unending, eternally prejudicial, unchanging, and immovable in your demeanor. You deliver cruel justice: premeditated, unforgiving, severe, relentless, and tenacious."*

- Most powerful mind of all types (and you know it)

- Always brave, courageous, assertive, never impulsive
- A slow mind with powerful brain capacity and potential
- Everything is under the control of your reason and thought
- Have caution and certainty; high ideals manifest in action
- You add up the facts (in your large left brain) and take action; you abhor inaction and laziness
- High potential in science, engineering, politics, speech, military, mathematics—anything objective
- You speak your truth energetically, arrogantly, forcefully, and honestly (if others do not like your attitude, too bad!)

▶ *While working in laboratory medicine with a calciferic research scientist, I noted that he would write his thoughts and commentary between the lines and along the margins of his textbooks. Each book was almost unreadable because of his writing. When I asked him a question, he would tell me the page number in a book that I needed to look at! An incredible memory.*

Potential Challenges

You may have evolved from, or not experienced these general faults, so do not dwell on them (not that you would).

▶ *If you relate to any of these challenges, doing something to overcome them serves your evolution.*

- Highly stubborn
- Cold, stern, uninviting
- Express feelings as felt
- Express anger with fists or tongue
- May be insensitive; easily drive people away
- Highly aggressive; bluntness may hurt others
- Readily condemn self and others for mistakes
- Vengeful, vindictive: never forget or forgive a hurt
- May be suspicious, gloomy, pessimistic, and cynical
- Argumentative, make enemies easily, lack diplomacy
- May over-indulge in alcohol; are not found drunk in public
- Cynical, skeptical, pessimistic, never defeated; you expect problems and are always prepared

▶ *A calciferic male I knew was a drug addict using cocaine and alcohol through the workday in his business without anyone realizing it.*

Calciferic Stress Management

Your strong *mental and emotional* stress prevention gives you a good ability not to internalize stress into your body. You would call the above challenges to be strengths.

Love

You are strong and passionate at the beginning of a relationship but the passion soon cools. A strong, highly-charged sexual drive and performance is always present. You have a dominating and intimidating chauvinism. You usually choose intelligent companions from the *carboferic, carbogenic, desmogenic, myogenic, nervimotive, and nitropheric* types.

Talents and Vocations

Abilities —*Academia, engineering, medical research, sports, science, mathematics, military*

Calciferic people are potentially brilliant and famous. You make great lawyers, scientists, inventors, engineers, mathematicians, speakers, executives, negotiators, motivators, and leaders of industry. The type information cannot predict what you will become, but the *calciferic* is capable of bringing a creative excellence or brilliance to whatever you do in life. You manage people with an iron fist, and expect respect for your mental power and leadership, but people rarely like you. You have the most creative brain in coming up with new ideas, methods and approaches for solving any problem.

▶ *I have known, or observed you, as actors, successful business people, scientists, restaurant owners, and as university professors. You are like a giant wheel: slow to start, hard to stop and filled with latent power. Most of us will never meet one of these people, but if you do, they are unforgettable!*

Inabilities —*The arts, music, diplomacy, political*

You are weak in artistic or diplomatic qualities.

———

Health Problems

You have great longevity, and if not diseased you may live very long.

▶ *Rocine: "Your diseases are associated with calcium deposition and hardening of tissues."*

In this regard, work with a nutritionist to remove environmental toxic metals and chemicals from your tissues: such toxins interfere with your calcium metabolism and health. If sick, you commonly experience health problems or diseases in any of these organs and tissues:

Stomach — You have an intense mind, and may hold mental stress in your stomach with ulcer vulnerability.

Pancreas — Excessive white sugar intake easily irritates this organ.

Heart, Kidneys, Lungs, Liver — These organs are vulnerable to disease from smoking, excessive dairy foods, and red meats.

Lymph — These small vessels are inefficient and sluggish (unlike the *hydripheric* who has an overactive lymph system).

Rocine wrote that with your strong mind, ego, and certainty of what is best for your health and well-being, you may well ignore most health advice, as it is very difficult for you to take advice from other people. I found in clinical practice that actors I knew, with their huge 'left' brains, were also able to embrace the 'right' brain aspects of their healing, and to have faith and trust in their healing.

▶ *Rocine: "Associated with your calcium deposition you precipitate sodium and chloride salts into your tissues, resulting in diminished respiratory function, pneumonia, lung, heart, liver, and kidney problems."*

———

Acid/Alkaline Factor

For your health and healing, the genetics of your autonomic nervous system predispose you to needing a specific ratio of food acidity to alkalinity. You are born with an *alkaline* constitution, which means you need a predominantly **acid-ash** food intake for acid/alkaline balance. (Ash refers to the minerals left in your body after metabolizing foods.) Your autonomic nervous system genetics are *parasympathetic* dominant. Theoretically, you need 70% acid-ash foods (proteins, carbohydrates) in your diet, but you eat them to excess and...

> *For your healing, if in ill health or after about age 40-45, you need to aim for this approximate ratio of food selections:*
> *50% Fruits, salads, vegetables*
> *50% Proteins, carbohydrates*

▶ *Approximate your food ratios. On any particular day, it does not matter if one meal is mostly alkaline and another mostly acid—just try to balance it out for the day! If you make a mistake, try again tomorrow. It is a subjective call that you make, and what is done over time that makes the difference to your health.*

The Calciferic Spiritual Factor

Skip this paragraph if uninterested in a philosophical perspective on your type!

▶ *Rocine: "The soul chooses the body type."*

If as souls, we choose the brain and body type to spend a lifetime in, it could be to learn certain spiritual lessons related to perfecting ourselves, and our humanity, in God's eyes.

What lessons does the type bring you? Only you can really decide what those lessons are. You know your weaknesses, faults, and behaviors towards others. You know things about yourself that Victor Rocine could never get from his research subjects when he first wrote about types. So search your mind for the answers. Each discrete type has challenges of life lessons, spiritual goals, etc., and some of yours may be:

Lack of Faith — You lack faith in anything outside of yourself; you benefit by nurturing a belief in God; and when, on occasion, you do embrace God, nothing ever shakes your belief. *[I knew a calciferic man who was a minister, author, scientist, and an esteemed international religious authority in his church.]*

Your faith is cerebral. You have a strong mental body, and you often conclude that believing in God is a stronger choice than not believing.

Unforgiving — You are vindictive and need to become more magnanimous, forgive others for not having your brilliance.

Impatience — You need to develop patience with those of inferior intellect.

Cold Demeanor — You need to cultivate friends not your equal, as your demeanor may drive potential friends away. Balance out your brilliance with being more human, kind, considerate, loving, and caring for those of us beneath your station, so to speak.

Argumentative — You make enemies easily because you lack tact and diplomacy; be kind to us mere mortals!

Arrogant, Aloof — You really are superior to others, but practice humility anyway! Consider that in God's eyes you are no better than anyone else. Developing humility seems to be a major lesson. Others see you as arrogant and ego-centric, but you know it is not arrogance when the knowledge you have **is** the truth! It is not that the rest of us are so dumb compared to you, but that few people have your brain inheritance. Accept us as having different genetics than you, and allow yourself to believe, we may know something that could enhance your knowledge, your healing, or your way of life.

[You may find the above aspects interesting, but inconsequential as to how you live your life and interact with others.]

———

A Calciferic Story...

John, age 46, 6'5, with a face carved from granite, had deep lines in his cheeks, sparkling blue eyes, a sturdy brain and physical frame, strong jaw and teeth, and a great white toupee marked him as the calcium type! His general health was good, but he had osteo-arthritis and daily back pain.

His diet was deficient in potassium and sodium foods: scallops, dulse, rice bran, strawberries, lobster, Swiss chard, beets and greens, celery, cod, sesame seeds. I advised him to eat two servings of these foods daily, and to stop using the salt shaker and taking calcium supplements; he also removed the high calcium foods from his diet: kelp, Swiss and cheddar cheese, almonds, parsley, corn tortillas, Brazil nuts, watercress, dried figs, and milk.

John also needed connective tissues supplements, particularly MSM and Chondroiten, which he took for several months. Over several weeks, his arthritic and back pains resolved, and he was soon pain free.

———

Calciferic Type Mineral Needs

Apply this mineral data to the diet following the Muscle type descriptions.

Excessive Foods:

- *Calcium*
- *Sodium (salted, junk food)*
- *Nitrogen (beef)*

Deficient Foods:

- *Potassium*
- *Sodium (unsalted, non-junk))*
- *Manganese*
- *Magnesium*
- *Nitrogen (non-beef, vegetable)*

*These deficient nutrients are common deficiencies in your type, and predispose you to ill-health.
If ill, be sure to use these lists with your daily food intake. If not ill, eat from the food lists 3-4 days weekly for health maintenance. All food lists are in descending order of concentration and value to you; choose servings of foods in the upper half of each list first! One serving is ½ cup.*

Calciferic Excessive Foods –

Calcium is excessive in your tissues. It is highly concentrated in the bones, joints, muscles, nerves, heart, teeth, and gums, and calcium excess is a significant problem in your illness or disease. (This often requires the help of a nutritional expert aware of how environmental toxicity interferes with your calcium metabolism.)

Sodium from salted junk foods is excessive in your tissues. To preserve your health and weight control you should avoid junk foods and fulfill your sodium needs from the food list (and lose the salt shaker). If you have illness or disease, restricting sodium from salt and salty foods is an important healing factor.

Nitrogen from red meat is excessive in your diet and a major cause of your acidity and illnesses; have it 1-2 times monthly if not ill.

Deficient foods -

In illness or disease, it is important to correct these mineral deficiencies.

Potassium is deficient in your type. It is concentrated in and vital to the health of your muscles, heart, brain and all cells. If you are ill or diseased, potassium foods and supplements may be a significant healing factor.

Sodium in its naturally occurring food form is deficient (see above note). Fulfill your sodium needs from the food list without using the salt shaker.

Manganese, often deficient in your tissues, is particularly needed in joint and muscle health; it is involved in critical enzyme reactions, and in bone, cartilage, disc, fat, protein, RNA, cholesterol, and carbohydrate metabolism.

Magnesium may be deficient in your type; it is particularly important for your heart, digestion, and metabolic functions.

Nitrogen, is needed from poultry, fish, and eggs (3-4 days weekly), with vegetarian proteins like legumes, peas, beans, seeds, nuts, and pasta on the other days. *[See the Appendix for notes on mineral functions and deficiency symptoms.]* _____

Minimize *Excessive Foods*

Calcium: *2-3 servings/week*

Swiss and cheddar cheese, turnip greens, almonds, brewer's yeast, parsley, corn tortillas, dandelion greens, Brazil nuts, watercress, dried figs, yogurt, milk, sunflower seeds, whole wheat.

Sodium (salted, junk):
0-1 servings/week

Salt, all fast foods, packaged foods, canned and frozen foods, soy sauce, all preserved meats (cured, smoked, canned and luncheon meats), sauces (barbecue, catsup, etc.), dill pickles, sauerkraut, bouillon cubes, peanut butter, potato chips, etc., salted nuts, crackers, canned or packaged soups, processed cheeses, commercial salad dressings, meat tenderizer. Note: If you must eat anything on the above list, keep it down to 0-1 times weekly!

Nitrogen (beef): *only 1-2 times monthly*

Beef, red meats (other than lamb)

<u>Eat</u>
Deficient Foods

Potassium, Sodium (unsalted):
1-2 servings/day

Scallops, dulse, rice bran, strawberries, lobster, Swiss chard, beets and greens, celery, cod, sesame seeds, turnips (not tops), dried prunes, peanuts, avocados, pecans, yams, parsnips, carrots, halibut, Chinese chestnuts.

Manganese: *1-2 servings/day*

Nuts (not Brazil), whole grains, legumes, rhubarb, Brussels sprouts, corn, cloves, rice bran, ginger, cabbage, walnuts, green tea, chives, peaches, alfalfa, eggs, endive.

Magnesium: *1-2 servings/day*

Cashews, blackstrap molasses, buckwheat, dulse, filberts, peanuts, millet, pecans, walnuts, rye, beet greens, coconut, Swiss chard, collard leaves, shrimp, sweet corn, avocado, prunes (dried)..

Eat...
Nitrogen (non-beef, vegetable):

Eggs, poultry, fish, lamb —3-5 days weekly
Legumes, peas, cabbage, black-eyed peas, seeds,
most nuts, pasta, spirulina, oranges, potatoes,
soybeans —as desired

Important Rocine Note

If unhealthy, Rocine recommended eating 1-3
servings of these two food categories daily:

Citric acid foods:

Grapefruit, citron, limes, oranges, pomegranate,
raspberries

Formic acid foods:

Avocado, cucumbers, mangos, pears,
persimmons, pineapples

If in good health be sure to eat these foods
regularly. The food recommendations are for the
generic type. Additionally, you may need from a
holistic healer or nutritionist something more
specific for your individuality.

Calciferic Nutritional Supplements

- **Potassium** — *[Take all supplements with food.] —99 mg/day*

- **Do not take Calcium or Multi-Minerals —**
  You have excessive calcium in your body.

- **MSM, Glucosamine and Chondroiten** — *500 mg/day*

- **Manganese** —
  50 mg/day (for connective tissues)

- **Herbs** —
  Brain detox – Gingko or Chamomile
  Organ detox – Saw Palmetto or Milk Thistle (Take one capsule, twice daily for s month; then three times weekly.)

- **Lecithin** —
  1,300 mg/three times weekly

- **Evening Primrose or Flaxseed Oil** —*1 soft-gel/day with food*

Important Calciferic Health Concerns

Your nervous system genetics require the *Muscle* type Food Guide for health, and any flesh cravings are normal and healthy for you. After age 40-45, you need a more *semi-vegetarian* diet with less flesh: about three flesh days and four vegetarian days per week.

CALCIFERIC FOOD GUIDE

Aim for -
50% Proteins, simple carbohydrates
50% Fruits, salads, vegetables
and
50% Raw food diet
50% Cooked foods

Eliminate all dairy foods, and the salt shaker!

Take the recommended supplements.

Weight Loss

Losing weight is relatively easy; follow the type instructions summarized in this section:

- *Stop* eating carbohydrates including all white table sugar and high-fructose corn syrup and drinks containing these sugars
- *Eat* your body type deficient mineral foods daily
- *Exercise*: your body type requires moderate to intense daily exercise
- *Calories:* As with any dietary approach, calories in must be *less than* calories out! Most markets sell a calorie booklet; make notes of your daily intake, and in most instances keep it under about 1500 calories/day

---

Muscle Types
General Food Guide

(Carnivores)

Important Note

———

The Food Guide addresses the <u>Acid-Alkaline</u> aspect of your food intake, along with the <u>Type Mineral</u> factor presented throughout this book. It does <u>not</u> necessarily address calories or other dietary factors that may be pertinent to your personal health needs whether medical or appropriate for some other dietary need. So use your common sense and just include the factors described here with whatever healthy dietary choices you usually make.

For other nutrient information, consult with nutritional books or with holistic nutritional doctors. I particularly recommend the advice of Andrew Weil, M.D.

———

General Food Guide

*This is a **general** Food Guide, upon which you superimpose the nutritional information from your type chapter. As a Muscle body type your genetics require flesh foods. (Note that a Thin sub-type would move you towards being semi-vegetarian.)*

Meat/Flesh Intake

Most muscle types should limit red meat to once or less weekly, while eggs, lamb, fish, or poultry are excellent in moderation. If ill or diseased, be sure to eat daily, one or two servings from each *deficient minerals* list. If not ill, eat them at least three times weekly for health maintenance. If this diet is similar to your present diet, but healing is sluggish, then:

- Decrease your carbohydrate and protein intake by about one-third
- Increase your fruit, salad, and vegetable intake by about one-third
- Consult with a holistic doctor, preferably one versed in nutritional and emotional evaluation

---

Over-Acid or Over-Alkaline?

Just as a log of wood burned in your fireplace leaves a mineral-ash, food ash refers to

the minerals remaining after metabolizing foods
in your tissues:

- Fruits and vegetables **alkalinize**
  tissues
- Proteins and carbohydrates **acidify**
  tissues

Usually You Are Over-Acid Due To:

- Excessive intake: dairy foods
- Excessive intake: proteins, carbohydrates
- Deficient intake: fruits, vegetables
- Accumulated metabolic waste-acids
  (from years of eating excessive meats
  and carbohydrates, and lack of exercise)
- Estimate the ratio of foods eaten.
  Generally, eat the following *approximate*
  ratio of foods for your health:

50% <u>Alkaline-ash</u> foods *(fruits, salads, vegetables)*

50% <u>Acid-ash</u> foods *(complex carbo-hydrates like starches, grains, cereals, breads, flour products; and proteins)*

Approximate your food ratios. On any particular day, it does not matter if one meal is mostly alkaline, and another mostly acid—just try to balance it out for the day! If you get it wrong, try again tomorrow. It is a subjective call that you make, and it is what you do over weeks, months, or years that make the difference—not on any one or two days or weeks.

———

Note - If Vegetarian

As a general indication, if you follow a vegetarian diet substitute vegetable sources of protein for the any flesh in the food guide. Note that contrary to most alkaline-ash vegetarian diets you need something different:

*You need an **acid-ash** vegetarian diet high in complex carbohydrates and vegetable proteins.*

Because of your high need for protein, you usually require a daily vegetable powdered protein supplement in juice (about 25-30 grams).

———

Important

- Minimize white sugar and alcohol intake.
- If desired, interchange lunches for dinners.

- Never eat foods you are allergic to, no matter what I recommend; if allergic, or suspect a food allergy, eliminate it and substitute from your type mineral lists.

- Eat the right foods 80-90% of the time and the Food Guide will work for you; unlike some types you do not have to live out of a health food store (although such foods are healthier for you).

▶ *Omit eating the excessive minerals in your type chapter, and be sure to eat one or two servings from the deficient list daily.*

Finally, in addition to your body type needs, other holistic healing matters also need your attention. I strongly suggest that you refer to my web site and earlier books for that information: *DrStenbeck.net*

———

Acid/Alkaline Genetics Chart

The following chart reflects each Muscle Type needs for acid or alkaline-ash foods. These ratios change if you are unhealthy or over age 45-50. Refer back to your body type and review the *Acid/alkaline* instructions.

———

Acid/Alkaline Genetics, Dietary-Ash, and Raw Food Needs

This chart shows the Rocine types, their acid or5 alkaline food needs, and the percentage of raw foods needed for your health and healing.

- Apply your Type Minerals to the Food Guide

Type Genetics	Acid/Alkaline Needed	% Food-Ash Needed	% Raw Food
Calciferic	Alkaline	50% acid	30
Carbogenic	Alkaline	50-50	50
Desmogenic	Alkaline	70% acid	50
Eldic	Intermediate	50-50	50
Medeic	Intermediate	50-50	50
Myogenic	Intermediate	50-50	50
Nervimotive	Alkaline	70% acid	50
Nitropheric	Acid	70% alkaline	70
Pallinomic	Alkaline	50-50	30

The above percentages vary depending on aging and the health of individual types.

Muscle Types Food Guide
<u>*Breakfast*</u>

Use the nutritional information from your Type Chapter everyday in this Guide.

EGGS* (1-2) with lettuce, tomato, or salad,   whole grain toast; (add bacon or sausage 1-3 times weekly if desired) — 2-4 times/week; or

FRUIT fresh salad, and protein (yogurt, milk, cheeses, seeds, nuts) —1-3 times/week; or

CEREALS, with fruit, seeds, nuts —2-5 times/week; or

OTHER choices — 0-1 times weekly

<u>*Daily liquids:*</u>
Pure water, citrus, vegetable juices, soups, other —as desired
Coffee, teas —0-2 cups

Lunch

SALADS, *mixed green, protein (poultry, fish, egg, cheese, seeds or nuts, etc.), whole grain breads*
[Dressing: olive oil/vinegar; low-fat, low-cal dressings]
— 2-4 times/week; or

SANDWICH, *whole grains with a protein (cheese, tuna, ham, etc.); and salad and/or vegetables*
— 1-4 times/week; or

POULTRY, FISH, *3-6 oz., with a mixed green salad and/or vegetables*
—1-3 times/week; or

OTHER *choices (with salad or vegetables)*
—1-2 times/week

[Other oils are permitted, but less ideal: soybean oil is a common allergen; minimize commercial dressings. Be sure to include two or more selections from your type food lists in your daily food intake. For in-between meal snacks, eat fruit or vegetables with seeds/nuts.]

Food Guide
Dinner

POULTRY, FISH *(4-6 oz.), with salad and/ or vegetables*
—2-4 times/week; or

PASTA *with protein (chicken, etc.) with salad and/ or vegetables*
— 2-4 times/week; or

VEGETARIAN *meal with salad and/ or vegetables*
—1-3 times/week; or

LEAN BEEF *(4-6 oz.) with salad and/ or vegetables*
— 0-1 times/week

OTHER *choices with salad and/ or vegetables*
— 0-1 times/week

Desserts:
Fruits, fresh —as desired
Low-sugar, healthy desserts
— 0-3 times/wk

Food Guide Notes

Steamed Vegetables —

Minerals are lost in the boiling of vegetables; steaming or wok cooking is best.

Food Combinations —

If you have a weak digestive system then eating proteins at the same meal with starches often results in indigestion, gas, or constipation.

Periodic Detox —

You tend to over-indulge in acid-ash foods (proteins and carbohydrates), and often need occasional elimination diets for tissue waste-acid removal. Have a holistic doctor or nutritionist supervise such detox (where you have an alkaline-ash diet along with protein supplementation).

Minimize —

- Fatty foods
- Commercial salad dressings
- Beef, red meats, processed meats
- Coffee, white sugar, corn syrup, alcohol

Vegetarian Proteins —

You require a carnivorous diet. The exception is the *nitropheric* type who functions best with a *vegetarian* diet; the other muscle types are born to be carnivores. It is very difficult for the other muscle types to be pure vegetarians because of their strong intuitive cravings for fish, poultry, meat, or eggs. If you are vegetarian, then because of your high needs for amino acids and acid-ash foods, you should take a protein supplement of 30-40 grams/day (powdered protein in juice).

Healthy Weight —

Several of you gain weight as the ravages of age, lack of exercise and dietary excesses take their toll. By eating according to your body type, you should naturally lose excess weight. Each type also has a few individual factors that only apply to them!

You have a good ability to lose weight by following the Food Guide instructions. The most common problem I find with your weight-control is liver and kidney irritation due to food allergies, which results in extra pounds. The key is to eat non-allergic foods.

If drinking more than 3-4 cups daily of coffee or tea, you may have a hypoglycemic problem (low blood sugar), which contributes to making fat, ill-health, and delayed healing. (Refer to the earlier books for help with this healing.)

In some *Fat* types like the lean or medium-sized (when young adults) *isogenic and pargenic*, you may be inclined to call them *Muscle* types: study them carefully to discern the differences.

* * *

Appendix

Brief Extracts from
<u>The 22 Unique Body Types</u>

Appendix A

Types
(Brief extract)

Type comes from 'typus' meaning an image or impression, the study of types being called typology.

▶ *Rocine: "A combination of mental and structural features is consistently found in people of the same type."*

Rocine wrote that all types are a mixture of positive and negative qualities. He based his work on the biochemical individuality of our *mineral* absorption and utilization. Of course, all minerals are absorbed, but he postulated that different types of people *selectively* absorb certain minerals, to a greater or lesser extent, requiring specific mineral foods for their enhanced health and healing.

▶ *The type information cannot predict what or who you will become, or how successful or not, but your type is capable of bringing a creative excellence to whatever you do in life. If your type has negative qualities that you disagree with, remember that they are only tendencies and may or may not manifest in you.*

This book enlarges on Rocine's premise (early 1900's), integrated with the later research of Herbert Sheldon, M.D., Ph.D., at Harvard University (1930's), along with my fifty years of observations and experience with this subject.

Comparing your shared physical (and sometimes psychological) descriptions with the Celebrity Lists further assists the identification of your type. It is not that you will look exactly like, or be a twin to, any particular celebrity. Look closely at a celebrity's features: face, profile, height, weight, head, etc. If you know something about their talents, beliefs, success and failure spheres, health and weight challenges, attitudes and behaviors, etc., then you get clues as to what your type may be.

————

Understanding Types and Sub-Types

Each of us has a clearly discernible dominant type. Visualize the celebrity examples from movies, politics, sports, the arts and public life, and try to identify with their physical features. Look for similar features, remembering that you will not recognize all attributes in yourself. You are not looking for your twin!

The sub-type issue is the main reason people of the same major type can look so different. Remember that a type description does not characterize you exactly, but depicts your individual variant of a type.

▶ *The type questionnaire pinpoints the major features of that type: if the celebrity examples are unhelpful, you may be an unusual variant (in which case ignore the celebrity issue and give yourself 7 points on Question 1).*

Minerals

Minerals are essential life nutrients that accelerate enzyme and chemical reactions and provide a basis for your body typing. Although found in all tissues, different minerals tend to be concentrated in certain organs, their presence or absence contributing to the healing of such tissues; e.g., zinc accelerates prostate healing; calcium and manganese promote bone, joint and connective tissue healing.

Specific foods nurture each type, some people needing meats for their health others needing a vegetarian diet. A high potassium diet nurtures one person, while another needs high sulfur, calcium, zinc, or another mineral.

Mineral Digestion and Absorption

Compared to vitamins, minerals are *difficult* to digest, absorb, and utilize. In people with strong digestive systems, this aspect may not be important. The following factors should be in place for optimal mineral metabolism:

1. Stomach Hydrochloric Acid Production
2. Parathyroid Hormone Balance
3. Organ Toxic Metal and Chemical Removal
   [See details in The 22 Unique Body Types.]

———

Total Body Healing

Note that from a holistic healing perspective, in addition to minerals and type information, the following healing factors are necessary:

> *Nutrient Balance*
> *Mental Balance*
> *Emotional Balance*
> *Spiritual Balance*
> *Detoxifying Integrity*

The above factors are all important to your total healing especially if you are interested in self-healing (see my earlier books).

———

Appendix B

Researchers
(Brief extract)

The predominant workers in this area of human individuality from around 1880's to the 1960's are Herbert Sheldon, M.D., Ph.D., Roger Williams, Ph.D., and Victor Rocine, D.Sc.

Much information on Sheldon's research exists on-line and in medical psychology libraries; for interested readers there are other lines of research published in the last century. This present book is primarily about Rocine's body types.

Herbert Sheldon M.D., Ph.D.

In contrast to Rocine, Sheldon at Harvard University in the 1930's was trained in the scientific method and did painstaking research and publishing on human individuality. In comparing his findings with Rocine's work, a direct putative correlation is visible.

Roger J. Williams, Ph.D.

Another significant researcher in human individuality is the renowned scientist and biochemist, Roger J. Williams. He demonstrated that different people have varying levels of nutrients, enzymes, and other metabolic chemicals in their bloodstreams.

▶ *Williams's research firmly expands on the premise of individual nutritional needs in human beings. If interested in his research, I highly recommend his book <u>Biochemial Individuality</u>.*

Victor Rocine, D.Sc.

Note that when a negative feature is indicated, say neurotic tendencies, all members of the type are <u>not</u> that way; it is a type tendency reported by Rocine.

Rocine studied type-related diseases finding links between mineral and dietary factors with individual types and their diseases. In each body type, one or more dominant minerals are preferentially absorbed and utilized over other minerals.

He recognized discrete body types from their physical appearance finding genetically based mineral dominance to be the determining feature. He also correlated their physical features with psychological characteristics.

———

Appendix C

Genetics, Types, and Diet
(Brief extract)

This section deals with how nervous system genetics helps determine your eating choices for health: you are either born to be a predominant meat eater, a partial or complete vegetarian, or something between the two. The genetic factor determining this dietary aspect is the *sympathetic and parasympathetic* components of your central nervous system. This represents a basic factor in eating for health.

This chapter helps you understand your dietary inheritance, although instinctively, you may already have arrived there!

- If born **sympathetic** dominant you are *genetically acid*, desiring a predominantly *vegetarian* diet for your health (about 70% fruit, salad, vegetables to 30% proteins and carbohydrates).

- If born **parasympathetic** dominant you are *genetically alkaline*, desiring a predominantly *carnivorous* diet for your health (about 70% proteins, carbohydrates to 30% fruits, salads, vegetables). Few of you ever choose to become vegetarian because of the difficulty in satisfying your protein needs without meats.

- If born ***intermediate*** dominant you may eat food groups with little concern for the acid/alkaline factor. However, after age 40, you need a semi-vegetarian diet for healthy eating.

———

Chart of Relative Nervous System Dominance

In the following Chart, if you relate to many of the symptoms on one side you probably have that nervous system dominance; relating to both sides indicates *Intermediate* dominance.

If Vegetarian (Over-acid) --
  Eat 70% fruits, salads, vegetables
  And 30% proteins, carbohydrates

If Carnivore (Over-alkaline) --
  Eat 70% proteins, carbohydrates
  And 30% fruits, salads, vegetables

If Intermediate --
  Eat 50:50 of acid and alkaline-ash foods

Make an *approximate* estimate of your daily acid and alkaline food intake (such ratios varying from type to type).

———

Symptoms of Relative Genetic Dominance

Vegetarians (Over-acid)	Carnivores (Over-alkaline)
Sympathetic Dominance	Parasympathetic Dominance
little or no flesh desire	desire flesh
easily constipated	rarely constipated
slow digestion	fast digestion
easily dehydrated	not dehydrated
strong thirst	low thirst
pale face	flushed face
high pulse after food	slow pulse after food
easy gag reflex	slow gag reflex
cool dry skin	moist warm skin
nervous stomach	calm stomach
little eyelid blinking	much blinking
nervous tendency	mostly calm
slower healing	faster healing
low oxygen-uptake	good oxygen-uptake
easily breathless	seldom breathless
insomnia common	sleep easier
few muscle cramps	some night cramps
calcium deposits rare	get calcium deposits

Appendix D

Help Identifying your Body Type with Dr. Stenbeck

If you desire help in identifying your body type, follow these instructions, and answer the questionnaire. For further information and fees, send me an email from page one of the website:

DrStenbeck.net

First name: _____

Country of birth: _____

Upload photos and send to the above website:

- Head and shoulders: front and side views

- Full body: front and side views

- Also 1-2 teenage views

- If possible, casual photos of mother, father, siblings

MY TYPE CLASS MAY BE: _____

   (Thin, Muscle, or Fat)

AGE   -   _____

HEIGHT   -   _____ feet/inches

MY WEIGHT -   _____ pounds

   Heaviest at age: _____

- Lightest as adult: _____

- Estimate age 15: _____

VISION - Excellent Average   Poor:

HAIR -   Natural color: _____

- Thin/thick? _____

- balding? _____

SKIN - Quality: _____

- History of acne, boils, other:

_____

_____

TEETH   - Strong   Weak   Dentures

- Cavity history: Many   Moderate   Few

MUSCLES - Strong   Average   Weak

Sports played _____

JOINTS   - Strong   Average   Weak

HEALTH - Childhood diseases?

_____

_____

- Adult diseases?

_____

AVERAGE DIET

- Beef _____ (times/week)

- Poultry _____ (times/week)

- Fish _____ (times/week)

- Eggs _____ (times/week)

- Water _____ (glasses/day):

- Vegetarian? Vegan? _____

- Other? _____

- Did your childhood diet differ? _____

The above will help me know who you are! I will send you a follow-up questionnaire for further help in identifying your body type.

Appendix E

On-line Health Consultation with Dr. Stenbeck

For further information, or to comment on this book, or to receive a response on any health issue from a holistic viewpoint, send an email inquiry from page one of my website:

DrStenbeck.net

Following that, I will suggest further healing needs, which we may pursue with an on-line consult.

———

Appendix F

Notes

See my book *The 22 Unique Body Types,* available at the usual online source, for further information and details on all of the 22 Types. The Appendix in that book has further information about:

Mineral Functions and Food Sources

Further Reading

www.ingramcontent.com/pod-product-compliance
Lightning Source LLC
Chambersburg PA
CBHW071225280526
45787CB00002B/811